The Moral And Religious Duty Of A

Chiropractor

D. D. Palmer

Kessinger Publishing's Rare Reprints

Thousands of Scarce and Hard-to-Find Books
on These and other Subjects!

- Americana
- Ancient Mysteries
- Animals
- Anthropology
- Architecture
- Arts
- Astrology
- Bibliographies
- Biographies & Memoirs
- Body, Mind & Spirit
- Business & Investing
- Children & Young Adult
- Collectibles
- Comparative Religions
- Crafts & Hobbies
- Earth Sciences
- Education
- Ephemera
- Fiction
- Folklore
- Geography
- Health & Diet
- History
- Hobbies & Leisure
- Humor
- Illustrated Books
- Language & Culture
- Law
- Life Sciences

- Literature
- Medicine & Pharmacy
- Metaphysical
- Music
- Mystery & Crime
- Mythology
- Natural History
- Outdoor & Nature
- Philosophy
- Poetry
- Political Science
- Science
- Psychiatry & Psychology
- Reference
- Religion & Spiritualism
- Rhetoric
- Sacred Books
- Science Fiction
- Science & Technology
- Self-Help
- Social Sciences
- Symbolism
- Theatre & Drama
- Theology
- Travel & Explorations
- War & Military
- Women
- Yoga
- *Plus Much More!*

We kindly invite you to view our catalog list at:
http://www.kessinger.net

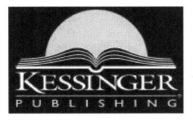

The Moral and Religious Duty
of a Chiropractor.

The following has been sharply criticised by a few chiropractors, but not as severely, nor by as many as was my announcement of the moving of joints by hand. A part of this criticism was based upon rival jealousy, the balance because of wrong impressions. That which was on account of a lack of information discontinued as soon as the would-be critics were well informed. I have received greater applause at the close of the following lecture from my classes than from any other. Every important chiropractic idea that I have advanced has been bitterly assailed, yet, although somewhat discouraged at times, I have not turned from that which I knew was correct.

The Constitution of the United States declares that "Congress shall make no law respecting an established religion, or prohibiting the free exercise thereof." The great state of California has granted the same privilege in its medical act, by declaring in Sec. 17, "Nor shall this act be construed so as to discriminate against . . . the practice of religion." It was quite mindful and generous of those who framed the California Medical Act to coincide with the Constitution of the United States in not allowing the Medical Act to conflict with the Constitution of the United States nor interfere with the religious duty of chiropractors, a privilege already conferred upon them. It now becomes us as chiropractors to assert our religious rights.

There could be no religion without science and philosophy.

Other states than California, in their laws to regulate the practice of medicine, have been mindful of religious conscience.

Kansas. "Nothing in this act shall be construed as interfering with any religious beliefs in the treatment of disease."

Virginia. "This act does not . . . interfere in any way with the practice of religion."

Washington. "This act does not apply to . . . nor interfere in anyway with the practice of religion."

Illinois. "Nothing in this act applies to . . . any person who administers to or treats the sick or suffering by mental or spiritual means without the use of any drug or material remedy."

The new law of 1913 of the state of California says, "Nor shall this act be construed so as to discriminate against . . . the practice of religion."

Chiropractic is a science and an art. The philosophy of chiropractic consists of the reasons given for the principles which compose the science and the movements which have to do with the art.

1

Science is accepted, accumulated knowledge, systematized and formulated with reference to the existence of general facts—the operation of general laws concerning one subject. Chiropractic is the name of a classified, indexed, knowledge of successive sense impressions of biology—the science of life—which science I created out of principles which have existed as long as the vertebrata.

Science is the knowledge of knowing. Scientific religion embraces a systematic knowledge of facts which can be verified by conscious cerebration. Knowledge is superior to faith and belief. Faith is an inward acceptance of some personal act; we believe thon is trustworthy, therefore, we have faith. Faith is a union of belief and trust. Belief is an intellectual process, the acceptance of some thing as true on other grounds than personal observation and experience. Faith implies a trust in a person. We may believe in a proposition in which no person is implied or thought of. Knowledge is knowing, we know from personal evidence. That which may be evidence to you may not be to me. That which we may accept as evidence today may not appeal to us as such tomorrow. Our belief, faith and knowledge depend upon our education. Our education depends upon our environments. Art relates to something to be done. Chiropractic art consists in the aptitude of adjusting displaced vertebrae, of which art I am the originator.

Chiropractic philosophy is the knowledge of the phenomena of life, as explained by the understanding of the principles, of the science and art. In my work on the Science, Art and Philosophy of Chiropractic I have given an extensive explanation of the laws of life and the nature of disease.

The practice of chiropractic includes a moral obligation and a religious duty. To comprehend these responsibilities it is absolutely necessary that the chiropractor should be able to understand and define chiropractic science. He must know not only the basic principle upon which it is founded and the constitutional parts which form its scientific structure, but, also, the philosophy of the science and art of vertebral adjusting. To absorb and digest these all important and essential ideas and make them a part of one's very being, requires a close study of The Chiropractor's Adjuster.

Chiropractic deals with biology. It is the only comprehensive system which answers the time-worn question "what is life."

Scientific chiropractors are versed in the principles of chiropractic. They live according to its rules. They philosophize on the art of relieving abnormal conditions by adjusting displaced bones. As Educated Intelligences, they relieve undue pressure on nerves in order that Innate may transmit and receive impulses to and from the various parts of the body in a normal manner. They desire to understand the nature of our physical existence and assign natural causes for both normal and abnormal functions.

As a science chiropractic explains local and general death to be but the result of law, a step on the road of eternal progression; that any deviation from tone, the basis of chiropractic, is disease.

As a philosophy it is the science of all sciences. It deals with subjective, ethical religion—the science which treats of the existence, character and attributes of God, the All-pervading Universal Intelligence. Its possibilities will become unlimited, when His laws and our duties as a segmented, personified, portion thereof, are scientifically understood. It will lessen disease, poverty and crime, empty our jails, penitentiaries and insane asylums and assist us to prepare for the existence beyond the transition called death. It explains why all persons are not equal, mentally and physically; or, if born alike, why some become superior or inferior to others similarly situated, why certain individuals are not able to express themselves as intelligently as others, why some persons are not mentally and physically alike at all times. To make clear this difference I will give a case and its termination under chiropractic adjusting. Ed., seventeen years of age, was hemiplegic in the left half of his body since birth. He had not uttered a word that was understood by his parents or friends. Mentally he was that of a child three years of age. Six weeks of chiropractic adjusting caused the distorted sixth dorsal articulation to become normal in shape and to occupy its normal position, releasing a stretched condition on the sixth pair of dorsal nerves, creating a normal tension of nerves and muscles, the usual force to impulses, arousing the normal amount of energy, consequently, the normal expression of ideas. In six weeks Ed's mentality and language was that of others of like age and environments. Conation (desire and volition)was equal to those of cognition and feeling. He became subject to the law of duty, capable of acting through his moral sense of right—he was a moral agent. He was, alike, intellectual in each of the three great divisions of the mind. I had performed a moral duty, as well as a religious duty. It points out the conditions upon which both health and disease depend. It explains why and how one person becomes affected with disease while his associate or neighobr, apparently living under the same conditions, remains well. Furthermore, it makes plain the reason why one, or more, of the bodily functions are performed in an excessive or in a deficient degree of frequency or intensity, either of which condition is a form of disease.

When Educated and Innate Intelligences are able to converse with each other, (a possibility which not a very distant future may disclose), we shall be able to make a correct diagnosis. Heretofore, these two intelligences have misunderstood each other concerning the laws which govern life. When the science of biology is correctly understood the span of life will be more than doubled.

Chiropractic has pulled aside the curtain of ignorance which obscured the cause of disease; in time it will lift the veil of superstition, which has obstructed our vision of the great beyond. In time, spiritual existence will be as well known and comprehended as that of the physical world.

Chiropractic science includes biology—the science of life—in this world, and the recognition of a spiritual existence in the next. The principles which

compose it are substantive in their independence and incentive to human
and spiritual progress. They originate in Divinity, the Universal Intelligence, and constitute the essential qualities of life which, having begun in
this world, are never ending.

It is an educational, scientific, religious system. It associates its practice,
belief and knowledge with that of religion. It imparts instruction relating
both to this world and the one to come. Supreme spiritual existence can only
be obtained through earthly experience. Chiropractic sheds enlightenment
upon physical life and spiritual existence, the latter being only a continuation of the former.

Chiropractic literature makes use of such technical terms as are calculated
to enlighten mankind in regard to the Universal Intelligence which the Christian world has seen fit to acknowledge as God. It enables its disciples to
recognize the above facts, and teaches them how to adjust their lives accordingly.

The casual thinker is obliged to admit that the universe is composed of
intelligence and matter; that the latter is neither intelligent nor creative,
while the former is omnipresent, filling all space; that this creative intelligence uses material substance for expression, and that life is the direct result of this intelligence seeking advancement toward perfection by the use of
visible, corporeal organisms.

Man is a dual entity, composed of intelligence and matter, spirit and
material, the immortal and mortal, the everlasting and the transient. The
manifestation of such an existence is intelligent action.

Chiropractors, especially, are aiding in this great advancement by adjusting the osseous structure, the position of which has to do with determining normal and abnormal tension, for in whatever part function is abnormally
performed tonicity is either lacking or excessive—Creative Intelligence is
prevented from expressing itself normally. Many a child has been injured
at birth by a vertebral displacement which caused an impingement upon one
or more of the spinal nerves, as they emanate from the spinal canal, the fibers
of which are distributed to certain organs. The result of this excessive tension is physical or mental debility, often both, which, from a lack of pathological knowledge, may be lifelong; the mental defect extending even into the next
world. For we retain only that which has been acquired during this earthly,
preparatory existence. By properly adjusting the neuroskeleton, these unfortunates may be enabled to acquire sufficient knowledge, rightfully due them,
to become useful members of society and enjoy life in this world and the one
to come. The chiropractor who can accomplish the above desirable results
and refuses to do so, as a religious duty, should be compelled to perform it as
a moral obligation.

Frank, a young man, twenty-one years of age, was brought to me for
correction. Physically, he was a cripple in upper and lower limbs. His
case was considered one of cerebral disease, an imbecile. An M. D. would

say, his diseased condition was congenital, acquired at the moment of birth, but, to a chiropractor it was acquired; in fact, all diseases are acquired, have their causes, whether before or after birth. In this case it was because of the sixth dorsal vertebra being displaced at birth. By daily adjusting the vertebra which had become abnormally shaped, was grown to the normal and placed in the usual position, thereby enabling the spirit to perform its desired avocation of creating a normal physical and the accumulating of normal ideas which will last throughout eternity. By so doing I was performing a service, a duty, I assumed when I accepted the trust bestowed upon me. By so doing I was not only performing a normal obligation, but, also, a (subjective) religious duty.

I hold it to be self-evident that all men and women who have acquired sufficient knowledge and skill to remove the nerve tension which prevents physical, mental and spiritual development, are engaged in a work of a higher order than that ordinarily required of, and performed by, the physician. They are practically the moral duties, and obligations of religion and any attempt to prevent such acts by law is an unmitigated crime against humanity.

Chiropractic science, its art and philosophy, deal with human and spiritual phenomena. The conscientious reverent acknowledgement of the phenomena, in sentiment and act, connects the spiritual with the physical, and constitutes in its fullest and highest sense a religion.

The knowledge and philosophy given me by Dr. Jim Atkinson, an intelligent spiritual being, together with explanations of phenomena, principles resolved from causes, effects, powers, laws and utility, appealed to my reason.

The method by which I obtained an explanation of certain physical phenomena, from an intelligence in the spiritual world, is known in biblical language as inspiration. In a great measure The Chiropractor's Adjuster was written under such spiritual promptings.

The object of a chiropractic education is the attainment of information concerning the origin, development, structure, and functions of our physical organism, the phenomena of physical earth-life and that of spiritual existence. These are acquired by observation and demonstration. Chiropractors declare that God is the All-pervading Intelligence, that each individual, segmented portion of spirit is a part of that intelligent creative principle; that only matter changes its form; that spirit modifies its environment, and dissolution is but a process of reproduction. Chiropractic science elucidates the problems of life, gives us the incentive to human endeavor and the agency by which sin, the violation, willfully or accidentally, of moral or natural laws, may be eradicated by appropriate adjustment of the neuroskeleton.

The cumulative function pertains to intellectual growth, whether sane or insane. As we retain our mentalities and carry with us to the great beyond only that which we mentally gather, it is necessary, in fact, it is a religious duty, to so care for our physical beings that our intellectual attainment may be of the very best.

The philosophy of chiropractic teaches the Universality of Intelligence and that its aim is always onward and upward toward perfection. This truth makes the practice of chiropractic a moral and a religious duty both in theory and in fact.

Religion may be objective in its character. As a cult it consists of the rites and ceremonies pertaining to the worship of a Deity, and only known by external, devotional acts of reverence. Subjective religion includes the moral and religious duty, the inner intellectual feeling, the science which treats of the existence, character and attributes of God and His laws regarding our duty toward Him. The former is that of theology; it includes the peculiar modes of divine worship which belong to and make the special distinction of tribes, nations and communities. The latter is ethical religion and deals only with positives, existing phenomena, properties which are knowable, together with their invariable relations of co-existence and succession. A belief in magic, the assistance of secret forces in nature, constitutes the essential of objective religion. The supernormal, the mysterious potency hidden from the understanding, the supernatural, the occult secret power, is the original, the basic element, the morbid outgrowth of subjective religion. Chiropractors deal only with moral obligations and subjective, ethical religion.

I do not propose to change chiropractic, either in its science, art or philosophy, into a religion. The moral and religious duty of a chiropractor are not synonomous with the science, art and philosophy of chiropractic. There is a vast difference between a theological religion and a religious duty; between the precepts and practices of religion and that of chiropractic. A person may be a conscientious devotee of any theological creed and yet be a strict, upright, exalted principled practitioner of chiropractic.

Chiro Religio, Chiropractic Religion, the Religion of Chiropractic and the Religious Duty of a Chiropractor are one and the same.

Willard Carver, D. C., asks, "Do you believe it wise to denominate chiropractic as a religion?" This question is equal to asking a physician, Do you believe it wise to denominate medicine (not the practice) as a religion?

Webster's Dictionary, latest edition, date 1910, gives near the bottom of page 1801, fifth column, the Latin phrase, religio medici, meaning, a physician's religion. Has not a chiropractor as much right to a religion as a practitioner of medicine? Is not chiro religio as consistent and comprehensible as religio medici?

"Do you believe it wise to denominate chiropractic as a religion?"

To denominate is to name, designate, specify or characterize. Wherein have I expressed a desire to RE-name the science, art and philosophy of chiropractic? In what sentence have I designated chiropractic by any other distinctive title than that by which it is now known? In what paragraph have I specified or characterized chiropractic as a religion? The science, art and philosophy of chiropractic is one thing: the moral and religious duty of a chiropractor is a different proposition. The founder, the fountain head, the creator, the originator, the developer, the one who named the science, art and philosophy of vertebral adjusting, says emphatically, it is not wise to denominate chiropractic by any other name or title than the one by which it is known the world over.

F. W. Carlin, D. C., writes me, "The Religion of Chiropractic is absurd."

I fully agree with Dr. Carlin. To say or think that the science, the art, or the philosophy of chiropractic, or that chiropractic, the three combined, has a religion, is really absurd and ridiculous.

He also says, "All religions are more or less based upon superstition. There is nothing superstitious about chiropractic."

He is right. All methods of treating diseases, as well as all forms of religion, are based upon superstition. Chiropractic as a science, as an art and the philosophy thereof, also, the moral and religious duty of chiropractors, are free of superstition, they are based upon the knowledge of principles and facts.

There is the moral and religious science of chiropractic, the moral and religious philosophy of chiropractic, the moral and religious responsibility attached to the practice of chiropractic, the moral and religious liberty granted to chiropractors by the Constitution of the United States; also, the moral theology of chiropractic, known in the California Medical Act as religion.

Morally, chiropractors are in duty bound to help humanity physically. Religiously, they are required to render spiritual service toward God, the Universal Intelligence, by relieving mankind of their fetters, adjusting the tension-frame of the nervous system, the physical lines of communication to and from the spirit. By so doing they greatly aid intellectual attainment and progress toward perfection through the untrammeled, mental reception of intelligent expressions of individual spirits. By correcting the skeletal frame the spirit is permitted to assume normal control, and produce normal expression.

The importance of bone-pressure on nerves as a disease producer (violation of public or divine law, the result of morbid conditions), is receiving attention by physicians.

The Los Angeles Times of May 25, 1911, gives a case of kleptomania wherein the knife was used to remove bone-pressure on nerves which were supposed to cause "criminal propensities." The "pretty 22-year-old woman, an uncontrollable kleptomaniac, had served one year in prison for shoplifting." The physicians considered her case "one of disease rather than of crime."

A month after the operation "a thorough revolution had taken place in her mental faculties. Her change for the good is going to be just as strongly pronounced as was her bent for the bad."

PASADENA, March 30.—Mrs. Jean Thurner of No. 315 West Avenue

50, Los Angeles, who attained almost world-wide fame two years ago when she underwent an operation for kleptomania at the American Hospital in Berkeley, at the hands of Dr. Herbert Rowell, who removed a piece of skull as large as a dollar from the top of the head, on the right side, was arrested at her home yesterday morning at the instigation of Detective Charles Betts, charged with the theft of diamonds and rings valued at $581 from three Pasadena jewelry stores.

Instead of using the knife and drugs, chiropractors substitute hand-adjustment of the displaced portion of the neuroskeleton which presses upon or against some portion of the nervous system, which injures, instead of protecting, the filamentous bands of nervous tissue that connect the parts of the nervous system with each other and transmit impulses to the various organs of the body.

The principles which form chiropractic science have always existed; and are now being revealed to the world by D. D. Palmer, through the Chiropractor's Adjuster. This revelation of the science, art and philosophy was given by one who tells me that he is indebted to those who are farther advanced in the knowledge of physical and spiritual phenomena than he is.

Through and by these discoveries chiropractors are able to relieve diseases which heretofore were pronounced by the medical profession as incurable. Thousands of cases of this kind can be cited.

I created a science out of the principles revealed to me and named it chiropractic. I correlated the art of adjusting displaced vertebrae together with the philosophy of the science and art. That these revelations were not made along the lines of medical and theological investigations is not strange when we consider that very few great discoveries have been made by those who were expecting results in certain smoothly worn grooves of stereotyped education. It is not surprising that those who have given to the world its greatest and grandest thoughts have been, more or less, connected with those who had passed into the spiritual existence.

Chiropractic gives relief to, and opens up a haven for, those who are ailing, making them physically, mentally and spiritually invigorated and whole. This noble work results in the direct salvation of countless numbers of mental and physical wrecks; for, the consequences of their disabilities do not stop at the grave, but continue on and on into the eternal spiritual existence.

An author on chiropractic states: "The special philosophy which he has worked out assigned as the foundation."

Philosophy, special or general, is not the foundation upon which I built the science of chiropractic. Its science is based on tone. Tone is the standard from which we note the variations of structure, temperature, tonicity, elasticity, renitency and tension; it is the standard of health; any deviation therefrom is disease. Tone is the BASIC PRINCIPLE, the one from which all other principles, which compose the science, have sprung.

Chiropractic is a science. The art of adjusting is the systematic, skillful application of chiropractic principles. Much study and correct reasoning upon the laws which constitute this science have developed its philosophy. The foundation of chiropractic does not consist of its philosophy, nor of the art of adjusting. I discovered the principles of which chiropractic science is constituted. By skill, directed by the knowledge of the science and its philosophy, I originated the art of adjusting. A knowledge of the science, art and philosophy of chiropractic contain a moral and a religious duty; morally, it serves as our basis of humane action according to our reason and judgment concerning our physical welfare; religiously, it governs our motives of divine duty with respect to the advancement of our spiritual existence throughout eternity. Its principles embrace the faith, belief, practice, obligations and conduct of our lives toward God and man.

Those who have a knowledge of, or a belief in, a future state of existence, regardless of church or creed, can become believers in and practitioners of, the religion OF chiropractors.

That which I named Innate (born with) is a segment of that Intelligence which fills the universe. This universal, All Wise, is metamerized, divided into metameres as needed by each individualized being. This somatome of the whole never sleeps, nor tires, recognizes neither darkness or distance, is not subject to material laws, bodily wants are not essential, substantial conditions are not needed for its existence. It continues to care for and direct the organic functions of the body as long as the soul holds body and spirit together.

Physicians deal with the physical only; chiropractors with both the physical and the spiritual.

Psycological investigation reveals the fact that the spirit of man is a part of the All Wise Spirit, the Great Creator, and as such possesses in an infinitesimal degree all the potentialities of omniscience and omnipotence existing in God, just as one drop of the ocean contains, in minature, all the qualities of the briny deep as a whole.

There are those who think the spirit of man has an abiding place in the solar plexus ,or in the spinal column, or in the medulla oblongata, or in the cerebellum, or in the cerebrum, or at least in some portion of the encephalon, but just what part or how much space occupied has not been determined.

The spirit holds the same relation to the body as God, the All Wise Intelligence does to the Universe. If you can locate the one, you can designate the location and define the limits of the other. God is indwelling in the universe, everywhere present; He occupies every part thereof; likewise, the spirit permeates every portion of the body in which it dwells. God does not depend upon the universe for His existence, neither does the spirit rely upon the body for its continued manifestations.

Although the surgeon cannot locate or dissect the spirit, that which creates intelligent action, yet we are conscious of this vital entity.

Knowledge of, or a belief in, the continuity of life has a tendency to uplift humanity, to make of man a desirable neighbor, a good citizen, a moral upright being and a practical understanding of right and wrong.

Innate is embodied as a personified part of Universal Intelligence, therefore, co-eternal with the all-creative force. This indwelling portion of the Eternal is in our care for improvement. The intellectual expansion of Innate is in proportion to the normal transmission of impulses over the nervous system; for this reason the body functions should be kept in the condition of tone. Communication with the Eternal Spirit, the Creator, is the goal of all religions.

There is no living religion without a doctrine; a doctrine, however elaborate, does not constitute a religion. The doctrine of our principles, faith and knowledge, are as follows:

I believe, in fact know, that the universe consists of Intelligence and Matter. This intelligence is known to the Christian world as God. As a spiritual intelligence it finds expression through the animal and vegetable creation, man being the highest manifestation. I believe that this Intelligence is segmented into as many parts as there are individual expressions of life; that spirit, whether considered as a whole or individually, is advancing upward and onward toward perfection; that in all animated nature this Intelligence is expressed through the nervous system, which is the means of communication to and from individualized spirit; that the condition known as TONE is the tension and firmness, the reniency and elasticity of tissue in a state of health, normal existence; that the mental and physical condition known as disease is a disordered state because of an unusual amount of tension above or below that of tone; that normal and abnormal amounts of strain or laxity are due to the position of the osseous framework, the neuroskeleton, which not only serves as a protector to the nervous system, but, also, as a regulator of tension; that Universal Intelligence, the Spirit as a whole or in its segmented parts, is eternal in its existence; that physiological disintegration and somatic death are changes of the material only; that the present and future make-up of individualized spirits depend upon the cumulative mental function which, like all other functions, is modified by the structural condition of the impulsive, transmitting, nervous system; that criminality is but the result of abnormal nervous tension; that our individualized, segmented spiritual entities carry with them into the future spiritual state that which has been mentally accumulated during our physical existence; that spiritual existence, like the physical, is progressive; that a correct understanding of these principles and the practice of them constitute the religion of chiropractic; that the existence and personal identity of individualized intelligences continue after the change known as death; that life in this world and the next is continuous—one of eternal progression.

"There is a natural body, and there is a spiritual body." 1 Cor. iv:44.

The spiritual and the physical are counterparts of each other, duplicates in form, shape, size and color. The evidence given by seers of every nation in all ages has been that a likeness exists between the creator and the created.

Locating the spirit in the brain, the encephalon, the mass of nervous matter contained within the brain-case, is circumscribed and yet not definite. The nervous mass within the cranium includes the two hemispheres of the cerebrum, the three divisions of the cerebellum, the pons varolii and medulla oblongata. Morphologically, these seven divisions of the encephalon are derived from the fore brain, the mid brain, the hind brain and the end brain.

The muscular, vascular and nervous systems permeate every avenue throughout the body. The conscious, characteristic actions of personified intelligence are performed through the nervous filaments of the body in which the spirit tabernacles.

The spiritual intelligence controls unintelligent matter through the nervous system. Each and every portion of the body is permeated by the spirit and its means of communication.

All functional acts are performed by the involuntary nerves; they direct organic life. The voluntary are those under the control of the human will, they look after the environments, that which supports and constitutes animal life.

There are two series of ganglia (nerve centers) lying along each side and to the front of the vertebral column, reaching from the occiput to the coccyx, fibers of which extend into the cranial, the thoracic, the abdominal and the pelvic cavities; these communicating nerve branches connect the vertebral chains to the various organs, vessels and viscera.

There are 144, or more, nerve centers, sympathetic nerve ganglia, designated by physiologists as so many brains differing in size, color, texture, functions, location, and more especially in the impulses received and distributed.

The controlling intelligence is everywhere present, manifesting through the nervous system its desires for advancement, making use of these nerve centers as receiving and distributing stations.

The founder of chiropractic has located the spirit in man, found its abiding place to be throughout the entire body, a position from which each and every nerve ganglia may be used for receiving and forwarding impulses.

Therefore, inasmuch as the light of life was revealed to me in order that I should enlighten the world, and as our physical health and the intellectual progress of the personified portion of the Universal Intelligence depend upon the proper alignment of the skeletal frame, I feel it my right and bounden duty to replace any displaced portion thereof, so that our physical and spiritual faculties may be fully and normally expressed, thereby not only enhancing our present condition, but making ourselves the better prepared to enter the next stage of existence to which this earthly existence is but a preliminary, a preparatory step.

By correcting these displacements of osseous tissue, the tension frame of the nervous system, I claim that I am rendering obedience, adoration and honor to the All-Wise Spiritual Intelligence, as well as a service to the segmented, individual portions thereof—a duty I owe to both God and mankind. In accordance with this aim and end, the Constitution of the United States and the statutes personal of California confer upon me and all persons of chiropractic faith the inalienable right to practice our religion without restraint or hindrance.

This is the end of this publication.

Any remaining blank pages are for our book binding
requirements and are blank on purpose.

To search thousands of interesting publications like this one,
please remember to visit our website at:

http://www.kessinger.net